GIVE IT NO THOUGHT
Know the Cause

Richard Grant

Solo the Clown
was with and without
wherever and whenever
without a doubt
happily contented
inside and out
he is whole
body and soul

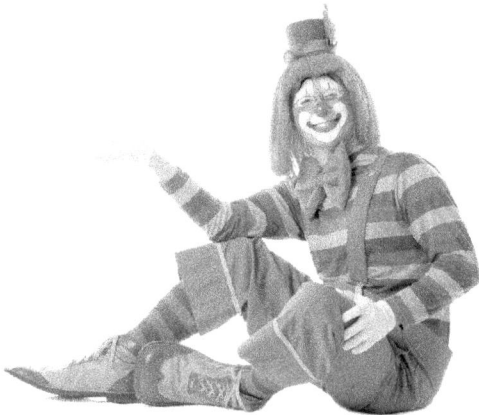

Acknowledgements

To Lao and Walter Russell, for setting up The University of Science and Philosophy at Waynesboro, Virginia USA. They have written many books, individually and collectively, most importantly the Home Study Course. (HSC) which have enabled me to come to grips with Who I Am.

Also I would like to acknowledge Glen Clarke for his book, The Man Who Tapped the Secrets of The Universe, which is a wonderful book about Walter Russell.

To unity School of Christianity

The Sermon on the Mount

Second Edition May 2011

Enquiries regarding any form of reproduction beyond the above permissions should be directed to the author:

Richard Grant
PO Box 735 Coffs Harbour NSW 2450 Australia
Ph: 0418 884816
Email: richardgrant15@yahoo.com.au
Website: www.giveitnothought.com
ISBN 978-0-9807030-0-9
Recommended Retail Price $20.00 AU

Every action is its own reaction, this means that when I perform any action I have already created its equal and opposite reaction.

Every thought has its own equal and opposite reaction.

To know the cause of how the material world is manifested, is to know how to heal the consciousness.

My senses perceive a sequence of events which are past and future, where there is no such thing

PREFACE

The purpose for writing this book is to bond with my inner self the awakening that I am experiencing as I let go all judgement, and to see with inner eyes only. In doing this I have come to understand the cause of how creation works, and this allows me to know the 'but why' of creation.

With this awakening I now know the body cannot experience sickness. My senses deceive me into believing the body is who I am, when in actual fact the body is only an expression of Richard. Knowing this, I can deal with the issues at the causal level of consciousness.

I feel this is how one man can change the world from within himself. As I practice this awakening in my everyday living, the quality of my life style has improved tremendously. This has a further effect on my friends and family around me who seem to have changed, when in reality I am the one that has made the change.

CHAPTER 1
THE AWAKENING

This whole book is about three words only - 'have no thought' - and the consequences.

I live on a 140 acre farm, with 100 head of cattle for company. My hours are from 'can see to can't see' (daylight till dark). Having no TV – radio – newspapers and no phone line, only a cell phone which is too expensive to use, my social life is limited. This has allowed me to live close to nature and to see the absolute inter-connectedness and the spirituality of all creation. I now know that 'everything that is, is of everything else that is'.

> *Have no thought to wearing glasses – the result,*
> *the eyes will adjust to all conditions.*

I spend a great deal of my time in bed pondering at night. Looking back at my life I realize what all my searching was about. I remember I was in Sydney for the first time when I was about twenty years old. I saw a tall man on the corner of the street singing out in a loud voice, 'I've found Jesus Christ'. As I had been searching for God myself for quite a while I approached him, tapped him on the shoulder and asked, 'Where did you find him?' He looked down at me with a look of utter contempt and refused to answer me, indicating that it was a stupid question.

Being a Scorpio I have an intense desire to know what causes things to happen - the 'but why'. I can remember as a small boy asking my father why was the bull on top of the cow? He replied, 'He's just looking at grass on the other side of the cow son'.

Who were those people out there that said, 'don't eat too much salt', and 'one must eat the crust on the bread to make ones hair grow curly'.

I went through the stage of trying to learn acceptance. I was into my second marriage and said to Elva my wife, 'You know Elva if you could just accept me just the way I am we could have a good marriage'. She replied, 'But you don't accept me'. 'What do mean I don't accept you?' I asked. 'You don't accept my non acceptance of you'. Oh boy, she had me there.

Have no thought of being tired – the result - you never feel tired.

I had a traumatic experience when I was fifty seven years old. Our son died of leukemia at the age of thirty four, leaving a wife and a three year old daughter. As I kept asking 'but why, but why did this happen?' it suddenly dawned on me that all the answers were within my own self. I had found God. It was like being reborn again, to know that God and Heaven are within my own self. Eternity is here and now. I now know that there is a spiritual universe, a 'temple not made with hands, eternal in the heavens' and that it can be discerned on this plane of existence but not with the human mind. This shift in consciousness occurred over twenty years ago, and since then I have come to know God as the creator of all there is. I AM that creator.

> *Have no thought of being cold*
> *the result - you do not feel cold.*

I no longer give my power away. In matters of health for example, I no longer put faith in green beans or carrots, or pills for sickness. I no longer fear death, old age, or any form of sickness. I am no longer held in the grip of fear in as much as taking precautions against it. Living in fear absorbs an enormous amount of effort plus energy which must be replaced by eating all the right foods and vitamins, which is a poor substitute for divine energy. As I give no thought to these things I have a feeling of peace and a clarity of mind.

> *Have no thought of mosquitoes biting you;*
> *where there is no fear there is no attack.*

Health is not a condition of body, but a condition of consciousness. Wealth is not a condition of purse, but of consciousness. I cannot experience freedom of my own. I cannot experience health of my own, nor can I experience wealth of my own. It is only in the degree that I experience the Christ consciousness, and the freedom of God made manifest as my experience, that I can understand the immortality of God the creator made manifest as my individual being.

Have no thoughts of aches and pains in the body,
they are symptoms only.

All beliefs lead to separation. As I let go of all my beliefs doors began to open - I saw that my beliefs were all fear based. It was always fear I gave my power to, which sapped my energy. I am at the point now where I would like to think there is no such word as belief at all. Living a life where nothing matters and having no thought, not even verbalizing thought, allows my true self to flow throughout my whole beingness.

The result of this is that I can now see with a clear mind many incidents that have helped me to let go of stuff I have been hanging onto.

For example, I had been working with Evelyn, helping her set up a spiritual retreat. I had become a vegetarian over a period of about four years and I mentioned to Evelyn that meat did not worry me any more. 'It does you know Richard.' she said. 'No I don't think about meat any more,' I answered back. 'You still talk about it so it must still be in your consciousness.' she retorted. I then had to concede she was right.

Have no thoughts to the results of no thought,
the result is a healthy body and clear mind.

Know that mind centers and controls motion from within, for it is written: '*Seek ye the kingdom of Heaven it is within*'.

It is in the *'letting go'* that I have experienced the most rapid awakening as I void each cycle of my life, knowing that I do not have to keep repeating my old ways.

Recently I was at a gathering of like-minded people when the topic of the ego was discussed at length. Everybody seemed to have a different idea of the word. Margaret, a friend of mine, wrote a whole page on the word ego. What she had written didn't sit well with me so I sat down and spent a couple of days trying to clarify in my own mind the meaning of judgment and ego. I eventually gave up when I realized there is no such thing as ego and judgment. They were all to do with the dream. *It was at this moment that I awoke to the dream.*

It is from that point that I now write the following awareness, looking at the universe from a totally different view point that has dramatically changed the way I live my life. I feel now that I have found the Christ within, where Heaven is. I have got to know Him, and now feel I can be God in expression. For God is mind in motion. I live in a mind and motion universe.

Have no thoughts for person, place or thing, everything just is.

Jesus the Christ was born in a manger, the most lowly of places. Just so is the Christ born in human thought, and that is about as low a place as we can reach in our individual experience. Why? Because all human thought is based on 'I' 'me' 'mine.' All human thought is based on getting, acquiring, achieving, and accomplishing. I feel this is the origin of the virgin birth concept.

As I have awakened to the dream I have come to realize that I live in two worlds simultaneously, the invisible universe and the visible (material world) universe. The invisible universe controls the visible universe, cause and effect. Each is one half of the cycle. The material world out there is a clear expression of my consciousness (invisible world) where I and the Father are One. For I am a clear pivot point of all that is.

For as much as God is the I AM of us, the I AM of us is God. I am not this body. I may have one, but apart from its service as a vehicle for the soul to gather experience it has no other value. Every person, place and thing I notice out there is a reflection created from within my imagination. The material world is mind in motion, which is God (mind) in motion. True perception is to see with inner eyes only, where everything is in perfect balance happening and un-happening simultaneously in the here and now where all is One. There can be no past or future. Eternity is here and now. I live in a perfect universe, where everything is an expression of itself.

Have no thought of seeing the differences, all is ONE.

A Guru visited his brother who was in an insane asylum, and his brother said, 'How come when I say I AM GOD, they say I am crazy and lock me up, and when you say it everyone follows you'. The Guru answered, 'Well the only difference is that when I say 'I AM GOD' I know everyone else is God too.'

Putting an end to judgment entails quite a shift. I realize that I must not see any part of the dream as having more value than any other part, there being no pairs of opposites in all creation. As long as I cling to any part of the illusion I am glued to the entire illusion, and vibrate at a low frequency, using up a lot of energy that is wasted, and the likelihood of a transcendence into light is virtually nil.

Waking to the dream does not mean everything disappears, it means everything appears as it really is. As I climb the mountain of life to a higher consciousness, leaving the valley far behind, I feel more alone. This aloneness that I experience gives me the opportunity to stand alone in my own power without the support of my fellow travelers. For I Am all there IS.

Have no thought to any beliefs, the result is there is no separation.

Without judgment there is no ego, fear, anger or resentment. Where there is no judgment I no longer see the differences in the material world. There is no more need to seek good health than to get rid of bad health; there is no more need to seek supply than run away from lack. There are no pairs of opposites out there. Everything is in perfect balance, for everything that happens un-happens simultaneously; each half of a cycle is seeking itself in the other half of the cycle in perfect balance at all times

If God is all there is, where guilt is not, forgiveness has no purpose and a state without a need for forgiveness must, of necessity, be a state of pure being, of innocence - a state of enlightenment. This in turn alters the frequency of the vibrations of the universe, which is God's frequency. This is what Jesus meant when he said that we can change the world from within. I then see all the material world out there vibrating as One, and this is a clear expression of my own consciousness allowing the abundance from within to flow freely. This in turn alters the vibration of my own self and the vibration of all those I come in contact with. Where we resonate as One and start to 'hum'.

Have no thought to a power outside of self.

For me to experience the past is to relive it here and now, and the same applies if I want to experience the future. I can only do that it in this moment, which is Eternity here and now. When I take judgment out of my life there is no need for acceptance. For there is nothing I can do to be. I, Richard, may see many problems out there but my true being can see no problem.

Separation from the oneness. To be kind and loving to another is not being, this is separation. To love another is to separate myself from my true beingness, which is to commit the primary sin. I then become the prodigal son - that is I separate myself from the 'Father and I Are One' and seek gratification in the illusion. This life is not about self gratification. The degree that I love another is the degree I do not love myself.

Have no thought to being positive, the result is you are never negative.

If somebody sees me as being judgmental, I am also judgmental.

Looking back in hindsight to some of the incidents I experienced in the past has helped me, knowing what I know now, allowing me to awaken more fully.

It was in 1995 at a spiritual retreat at a place called Rumbalara where we were gathered in a big circle at the end of a intense weekend workshop, and we were sharing with one another before going home. A lady on the opposite side of the circle stood up and burst into tears, saying what a terrible world we live in. I immediately jumped up and said, 'Oh no it's a wonderful world we live in', A lady called Joy on the other side said, 'Richard, now that's a judgment, and now I am judging you. Oh my goodness,' then sat down, realizing she was also judging. As I take judgment out of my life it seems to have a further effect, further effect, and so on.

Have no thought to old age, there is no such thing.

As I void the cycle of the dream I have a strong feeling I am awakening to something far greater than myself, for my eyes have been blinded for so long. I now know what I have sought for so desperately on the highways and byways of life. I must now learn to lose my own self in order to find my Universal Self.

When the heart weeps for what it has lost, the souls smiles for what it has found.

The word *I* is not a singular word, it is an all inclusive word, meaning 'all there is'. The soul has come home – for it is born anew – it is at peace – it is free. There are no two things in the universe, everything is expressing itself.

Have no thought to death, there is no such thing.

To know the truth will set me free, for there is only one truth and that is 'the Father and I are ONE. Know there is nothing out there. I cannot 'know' anything that I can see, feel, or touch. But I can know God, the creator of it. Knowledge of the nature of God will come through science, not through religion, and will set me free. So I give no thought to anything out there, my thoughts are the ego in motion. If I was a sparrow in the field with no thought I would be everybody and everything.

'Man is forever seeking the Light to guide him on that long, tortuous road which leads from his body's jungle to the mountain top of his awakening Soul. Man is forever finding that Light and is being forever transformed as he finds it, and as he finds it he gradually finds the Self, which is the Light. And as he becomes more and more transformed by the God Light of the awakening Self within him, he leaves the jungle further behind him in the dark from which he is being released by his gradual transformation from the electrical awareness of the Spirit. ... W Russell

The Father-Mother of creation divides His sexless unity into sex – divided pairs of opposites such as plus and minus, hot and cold, dark and light and so on, for the purpose of uniting them to create other pairs of father and mother bodies in eternal sequence forever.

As I ponder and comprehend that creation is a division of The Eternal ONE into countless two's of sex-conditioned opposites, which eternally seek to void their division by uniting as ONE.

Have no thought to being healthy, you are never unhealthy.

By following the one basic law of creation, that is the rhythmic balanced interchange between opposites, all creation emerges from its Creator and then returns to the Creator. This is an imagined mind and motion universe. What begins and ends is mere appearance. Life is a process of continual change; nothing (no thing) lasts. For everything that happens, un-happens simultaneously.

Have no thought to needs and wants, they are all false.

I visited Sai Baba in India in 1990 and experienced an enormous shift in consciousness. It was on the flight out of Madras that I heard a voice coming from within me that shouted, 'Know Who You Are'. I now know who I Am, God the creator. For I sit in the grand puppeteers seat. The only difference here is that I am the author, scriptwriter, director, actor, and audience all in one, where I create the play of life. All the characters in the play are also God, each being a clear expression of my consciousness, which manifested as the play of life, what used to be called the material world. For each incident and actor in the play I have created for a purpose, and so know who I AM. Even to the victims of the earthquakes that destroy thousands of bodies, I know that each soul comes into a body for the one purpose - to experience that trauma.

Have no thought to what goes into mouth,
only what comes out of it.

As I understand the cause of creation, I have the knowledge to know the purpose of all that happens. All traumas in life are blessings, it is only through suffering can I awaken to who I AM. I am of the opinion that I already have chosen my date of departure from this dimension, and there is nothing I can do about it.

Any thought of the body and its welfare will only cause separation, for the body is being cared for and maintained by the creator of it

Aches and pain in the body are thoughts in motion, use the mind to stop the thought, where there is no motion there can be no pain.

It is the thought that keeps the belief in motion, use the mind to let go of the thought, by giving it no more thought.

CHAPTER 2
THE LAW OF BALANCE

The key to good health is to be balanced.

To stay balanced one must stay centered.

To stay centered is to have no thought for person, place or thing.

To have no thought is to see no differences in creation, is to have no beliefs.

To see no differences is to know all is One.

To know all is One is to know all creation is an expression of itself, for I and the Father are One.

I have a deep inner knowing that I am pure consciousness.

To have this inner knowing is a powerful tool to healing the world.

There is one inviolate law running throughout creation that gives apparent time and motion: that is, *The Rhythmic Balanced Interchange between opposites.* It is the play of life, where each half of a cycle is trying to find itself in the other half of the cycle - like seeking like.

All of creation is made up of vibrations which we call cycles, and all cycles have an operating frequency (pulsation) normally of a number of times per second. For example, as I breathe in I compress, as I breathe out I express. This is one cycle. All cycles are either compressing or decompressing. The in breath (compressing) is the growing half, and the out-breath (decompressing) is the cycle coming to rest (living and dying). One of the hardest things for me to grasp is that what I see in the material world is only one half of the cycle. This is what I form my judgments on, not realizing what caused what I am judging.

The perpetuity of creation is based upon the constant giving of one half of a cycle to the other half for the purpose of repeating the creative process through another cycle of giving for re-giving. ... W Russell

The law of balance is also the law of love, for the more balanced one is the more love one is. This universe is founded on love as manifested in the giving of one opposite to the other for re-giving to the other. Whatever is true of God's universal body is true of man's body. It is the equality of balance between the giving and re-giving of Nature which makes its transaction perpetual. This is the play of life, which makes up the dream. Such divisions into halves are male and female – buyer and seller – positive and negative – compression and expansion, and countless other divisions of ideas.

For every action there will always be an equal and opposite reaction created simultaneously in the unseen world that I am not aware of. It's like walking a tight rope, continually being aware that balancing is taking place at all times.

Have no thought to any problem.

Having awakened to the dream, I now live my life where there is no judgment, ego, forgivingness or duality, giving no thought or reason to the outcome of my expression; as I chop wood and carry water (my daily chores) staying as close as possible to the center of my being, in the oneness, allows my life to flow freely, this in turn allows the reflections of my imagination to flow freely also, (the material world). Also, as I to come to grips with the fact my abundant supply of all there is comes from within the Oneness, eliminating all my needs and wants, I need never worry again about anything. I now know my body is being maintained and sustained by the infinite Consciousness that formed it, the divine consciousness of my being, and I am eternally being fed, not three time a day, but twenty-four hours of every day, from within.

The surest way to prevent me from getting anything for myself is to seek it for my own personal gain.

I have meat to eat that you not know of. But whosoever drinketh of the water that I shall give him shall never thirst; but the water that I shall give him shall be in a well of water springing up into everlasting life... the words that I speak unto you are, spirit, and they are life. ...John 8;32

Christ consciousness is that state of consciousness which no longer reacts to things in the outer realm. Nothing external – nothing existing as effect – can have power or jurisdiction over me

(Richard). There is nothing that exists as person, place or thing, circumstance or condition imbued with the power for good or evil. It is impossible for this body to suffer any form of pain, discomfort or illness unless I allow it or create it.

Have no thoughts to healing the body – result, a healthy body.

As I let go and let God, with no more thought, this balances the inner world of cause with the outer world of effect. There is only one power, one creator. I AM that law unto every effect. That what I would call sin or evil are but experiences where two unbalanced conditions fail to demonstrate the law of balance by interchanging their two opposed conditions equally. This blocks the flow of life where toxins build up, which eventually shuts life down. When I hate I am invoking the law and when I love I am invoking the law, when I give or share I am invoking the law, just as when I hold onto things. As soon as I begin to accept the principle that there is neither good nor evil in person, thing, or condition, this leads to living a life by grace.

When I seek abundance to fill a lack in my life, all I do is create more abundance of lack.

All suffering is created in thought, I must stop looking to thought for an answer

Which of you by taking thought can add to his stature one cubit, or can make one hair black or white.

All human thought is based on getting – acquiring – achieving and accomplishing.

It's my reactions to the world that guide me on my way

CHAPTER 3
THE VOIDENCE PRINCIPLE

We live in a thought wave, mirror imaged universe, made up of cycles of motion.

It has been a big help for me to understand the how and the why of cycles (vibrations). Each cycle in itself is a complete lifetime; it is born, lives and dies. As I breathe in I live, as I breathe out I die. This is one cycle, each becomes the other. As I work through the day I am expressing and creating for half the cycle. I then lay the body down at night to void the day's activities and recharge the body to complete the cycle. As I let go each cycle completely I experience a new beginning.

I feel now I have voided the cycle of the dream; it's as though a cycle of my life has ended completely and this allows the next stage of my awakening to unfold, where I now live in the world within, where there is no judgment. As I let the dream go completely doors are opening rapidly to a whole new way of living. Where I see a clear reflection of who I AM in a clear expression of my imagination which is expressed in the material world out there.

This is proving to be a wonderful tool for me to see issues in my life that I need to let go of. For the issues and problems I see out there which were created with my thoughts and judgments are a reflection of my imagination, which I have experienced, and if I don't like what I see, I know that I created it and I can change my way of living from within my own consciousness. I can change with inner thinking, working with God, for God will work with me but not *for* me. I see with inner eyes only. This in turn changes the world out there.

Have no thoughts because thoughts use up a lot of energy.

Dave and Mabel lived way back in the mountains and never saw much of civilization. One day Dave found an old mirror it the barn, and he had never seen a mirror before. He took one look in the mirror and cried out, 'Oh my God it's me father come back'. So he hid the mirror from Mabel. When he went out she found the mirror and when she looked at she exclaimed, ' If this is the old hag he is seeing I have nothing to worry about'. (the mirror effect of creation)

Dealing with issues out there at this level of inner awareness overcomes the issues that I encounter, so they do not occur again. There is nothing out there in the material world that can alter my vibrations or bring me down or lift me up that I have not created myself. For me to love something or somebody out there is to devalue who I Am. Everything starts within me and finishes within me. What I am dealing with out there is my creation, which is a expression of my own imagination. It is impossible to learn how to awaken: also it is impossible to teach how to awaken. For it's in the letting go of the old ways that I awaken to Who I AM. And so void the cycle.

The inner mind (God) is the only energy force in the world, on the condition I create from within the oneness, where I create with God. For God is mind.

To create on the outer with my thoughts, this is the ego's tool. Where my vibrations are of a low frequency I build on sand and am controlled by my senses and the ego which deceive me. On top of that, all my material world is only an expression of my own imagination. So it is important to be aware of the thoughts I hold in my consciousness. While ever I hold thoughts in mind, this takes energy from within me to give those thoughts motion, and this in turn supplies energy to keep those old beliefs, fears and judgments alive and in motion, because it's these thoughts that are reflected into the material world of my daily life. Thoughts are things; they are mind in motion, the ego. They create perceptions which are reflections, also they create beliefs which are fear based. If I have any fear I empower fear, and what I empower I attract. To fear I would have to fear myself.

Have no thoughts of things in the material world.

I feel it's the thought (belief) of the food that actually puts the weight on the body, not the food itself. It's the thought (belief) of the sun shining on the body that creates the cancer, so give it no thought. It's the thought of the mosquito bite that creates the sting.

It's the fear of not having enough to eat that creates the starvation in the world today, not the shortage of food. I feel it's the fear of death that kills the thirsty man, not the lack of water. I feel now it's so important for me to realize that when I give thought to what I have imagined I put that thought in motion, which gives us apparent time and motion.

Have no thought to trying to change person, place or thing.

The next step, which is one of the most important lesson to learn of all, is to give no more thought to what I have created - the cycle has finished, so I re-give what I have created back to the Oneness, where I have no attachments or value to what has been created. *Having no thoughts voids the cycle.*

To judge something is to give it thought. This in turn separates me from the Oneness. Even to put a name to anything is to judge it. This is the primary sin, and all suffering follows from this separation. The more attention I give to what I have judged or given thought to or verbalized, the greater will be its power to manifest, for what I am seeing is already created.

Having no thought is to give in.

I now notice that when I am with a group of people where there is no judgment, there is an allowing and bonding taking place. Where I observe myself without thought or judgment this creates a vibration which resonates at a common frequency, and we seem to become more as one with each other. As I see myself in everybody else, I would see this as my true beingness shining through, truth vibrating with truth.

To take this to the next step is for me to realize that everything in creation is a clear reflection of where I am at with my imagination. This includes, wars, suffering, sickness, ego. Every person place or thing is my creation - an image of my consciousness. Everybody is where I am at; if I see somebody who 'hasn't got it yet' it means I am the one who has not got it yet.

Have no thought to a healthy body.

Therefore to give something no thought is to allow my true beingness to shine through, for this is who I truly am - that childlike being that never ages but which is held down by all the traumas of living my everyday life. When something is voided it's as though it never was.

When hydrogen and oxygen combine to form water, there is no oxygen or hydrogen in the water. Death gives to life that it may live, and life gives to death that it may die. There is no such thing as death, nor is any such thing as old age. This body of Richard is only an idea of who Richard is, therefore the body has never lived, only the idea has appeared to live. For what has never lived can never die. What seems as death is birth, and so constant change the only permanence. I must learn that the giving half of the cycle must precede the re-giving. As l learn Nature's law of love and give of myself to my fullest extent, the law will unfailingly work to re-give in equal measure that which I have given.

I am not one, I am all men – billions of them. I exist in them and they in me. Whatever I think or do individually I am doing universally. My thoughts are everyman's thoughts, and theirs are mine. Every happening anywhere by any man or other body in Nature, simultaneously happens everywhere *throughout the universe, but each happening in any body informs all other bodies of a new condition of effect at a light speed of 186,400 miles per second.*

The world in which we live is a world of imagination

If a man's concept of himself were different everything in his world would be different. His concept of himself being what is, everything in his world must be as it is.

My reactions will tell my true state of consciousness

~26~

CHAPTER 4
THE MIRROR EFFECT

I live in a mirror imaged thought wave universe where I and the Father are One. The reflection of a light in a mirror is actually within the mirror. All creation is a mirror which reflects itself within itself universally. When I get up in the morning and look at myself in the mirror, I see a reflection of what my physical body looks like. If I want to have a look at my consciousness, my true beingness, I can see it reflected in the material world around me. mind knows and projects its light, senses can but sense motion and can never know cause. This reminds me of a yarn.

To have no thought is to eliminate sickness.

The husband came late one night drunk, and as he crept up the stairs trying not wake his wife he fell backwards down the stairway, breaking the bottle of whisky in his hip pocket and cutting his backside in the fall. He cleaned up the mess so that his wife would not know he came home drunk, putting band aids on his bum to stop the bleeding. In the morning his wife said,

'You came home drunk last night and fell and broke your bottle of whisky cutting yourself on the backside didn't you?'

'How do you know I cut myself?' He asked.

'Go and have a look at the band aids stuck to the mirror', she replied.

To have no fear is to be in Love.

All is Self, all is myself.

To see myself in everybody and everybody in myself is Love.

The world has no existence apart from Who I Am. At every moment it is a reflection of myself. I create it and I destroy it. Everybody I see out there is where I am at. I AM a divine immortal invisible soul centered in a physical body made up of thought waves of motion, this body I call Richard, who is never created. Only the idea of Richard is created. Having awakened to the dream I now see the whole universe as being a clear expression of my imagination. I create the puppets, but I am not the puppets. I AM the puppeteer.

Have no thought to what is right or wrong,
for one balances the other.

All action in creation is forever disappearing into a mirror of its own image of equal potential. There are no balanced opposites, as there are no two things in the whole universe, all is one, each reflecting itself in the other. Every person, place, or thing in the universe is God (mind) in motion, which is a clear reflection of my imagination. Seeing is electric sensing. Motion can sense only motion. They cannot sense the stillness of eternal balance. They can but sense the motion of divided balance. This is the purpose of my senses - to tell me when I am separate from the Oneness. It is like the rocket going to the moon, the gyroscopes tell when the rocket is off course. My senses are my gyroscopes.

Have no thought to being hungry.

Matter is but a mirror which reflects qualities outside itself to simulate qualities within itself. There is no knowledge, energy, life, truth, intelligence or thought in the motion which matter is. All energy is at right angles to motion, in the stillness at the center of the shaft - the fulcrum, as in a crank shaft of an engine. It is in the stillness at the center where God is, centering and controlling all motion. The same as the cyclone, God is at the center of the cyclone centering it. The same would apply to my body of motion, God is at the center of my being, balancing and controlling my every move. All motion is a continuous two-way journey in opposite directions between two destinations, happening and un-happening simultaneously. Every action creates its own equal and opposite reaction simultaneously.

Every effect of motion is voided as it occurs, is recorded (in its inert gases) as it is voided, and repeated as it is recorded. This gives the effect of time and motion, where there is no such thing.

There can be no conflict in the world, for it is within man himself. I must learn to look on matter – the material world, as a transient motion picture record of the idea which it simulates and which I have created, for that is what it really is - a cosmic cinema thrown upon the majestic screen of space. I must not for one moment forget the reality of mind nor the illusion of matter. As I transcend the world of body sensing, to the world of inner knowing I see with inner eyes only.

I realize that I am dealing with thought wave patterns of ideas, and not with substance or matter. Consciousness is all there is.

Have no thought to being thirsty.

For me to deal with any issue out there I would only be dealing with a reflection. It would be like I was trying to fix my face up in the reflection in the mirror. So looking at problems out there takes on a whole new dimension, because what I am seeing is only a reflection of my own imagination. I am forever looking at a mirror image of my own creations. If I notice somebody out there, I see them as a true reflection of my own self which is in perfect balance with my consciousness – the One mind – God. All is perfect.

Have no thought for duality, it is only a temporary state.

If I had a symptom appear in the body, my first reaction would be to know that it is impossible for the body to suffer any form of illness, then give the symptom no thought. What I am experiencing is a reflection of the cause which has been manifested in my consciousness by separation from the Oneness, which is the primary cause of all suffering, so I must deal with it at this level, the cause, and give no thought or judgment whatsoever to the ailment in the body. To do so would empower the symptom, (the symptom is not a sickness) for my body is also only a reflection of my imagination in the same way as my material world is only symptom of an inner cause.

Have no thought of 'I and mine', they are false ideas.

I can now see and understand what Jesus said, 'Even the least among you can do as I have done, and much more'. I have always been of the opinion that to change the world out there, human nature would have to change. I now know how to change human nature from within my own beingness. I can let go of the dream and see the reflection out there without judgment, ego and all the old ways of living out there, and live from within as One with the creator. All I have to do is to change the reflection from within myself. As I practice dealing with issues from within, seeing them as a reflection of my imagination, the people I come in contact will appear to have changed. In actual fact I am the one that has changed. It is only mind power, not technological power nor anything else that can prevent our present civilization from falling into oblivion.

Man is mind...Man is matter in motion...mind and matter are One...God is mind.

To know how to think in light from within is to open the doors of all knowledge, which is to know cause. There is no power in this universe other than the energy of inner thinking mind.

I have a friend who has just been assessed as have short term cancer, and this has caused me some concern. My talks with her indicate to me that she has some deep seated issues within her consciousness that she needs to address and let go of. Her sister's name comes up often, and I pick up there is anger and resentment coming from her when she tells me what sort of person her sister is. As I ponder this I now realize what I am seeing in her is a reflection of my own imagination, showing me that I have issues within my own self that I must deal with, that are fear based. As I eliminate my judgment of her and shift my awareness back to my inner self and deal with the issues from within, she will appear to have changed. This is the illusive part, for it is I who will have changed.

Have no thought for the body, there is no such thing, it is just imagined.

What I am seeing in her is an issue that I need to resolve within my own consciousness, this being a mirror reflection of something that is deep seated within my consciousness. Any thing I see out there reflecting back to me would have a fear base. It is impossible for me to attract anything into my life - I *create* everything. There is no such thing as the law of attraction except in the material world, this is one of the tools which the ego uses.

Have no thought what is conceived of the mind.

When I share with a group of like minded people now, all

coming from different

levels of consciousness with a different basic philosophy to me, I enjoy seeing myself in each of the others. The issues they bring up that push my buttons, I deal with from within myself. This enables me to let my old ways go and open up to a whole new way of seeing my fellow man change his ways. Ha ha, but it's me that has made the shift, so voiding the cycle.

I feel this is what Jesus was talking about. It is coming back to working with God at the level of Oneness from within. It is at this level where the shift will take place in the world, for the universe is within me. This means I now know how to make that shift that will change the world out there. To heal the world I first must heal myself. Knowing how to do this is so important.

The first step to change my consciousness is to let go all judgement – the next give no thought to whats out there. This eliminates blame.

To heal the world one must heal oneself, for the world is within man

It is impossible for me to see other than the contents of my own consciousness

This universe of seeming motion does not exist, my senses deceive me.

CHAPTER 5
HAVING NO THOUGHT

God is no thing ----------- God is no body

I Am no thing ------------ I Am no body

But if I was a sparrow in the field with no thought, I would be everybody and everything. For me to be somebody, I need to be nobody.

Thoughts put motions to words to create things. Thoughts and words create judgment, which leads to beliefs, all having a fear base, and this lowers the frequency of the vibrations thus blocking the flow of life and not allowing life to flow freely. Living this way uses up a lot of energy that needs replacing.

This is a path of self destruction. So have no thought, for thoughts are things - thought is matter in motion, thought is ego. To give something thought is to give it power to manifest. If I notice the weeds in the garden I give them power to grow faster. If I notice something about my body - what I will wear, my health, they all take energy. To take this a step further, it is my thoughts that are destroying my body, the same as when I try and save the world my thoughts will be the driving force that speeds the destruction.

Have no thought of working.

To have a healthy body has got nothing to with the body, it is all to do with consciousness. It is important that it has no baggage such as beliefs, fear, possessions, diets, worry, ego. The body needs to be a clear channel for consciousness to flow, for good health is a state of consciousness, not a healthy body. A healthy consciousness creates a healthy body. My aim is to live in a state of pure consciousness. If I am able to do this, then everybody else would be in that state too.

Have no thought of your bank balance.

The energy for this power comes from within oneself. I have found the less energy I give to anything out there the more energy I have to express with. He (Jesus) also said that thoughts are much more powerful than the actions of those thoughts. Thoughts use up a lot of energy, for they are the primary sin of separation. Thoughts set energy in motion, where in actual fact there is no motion. So if I give no thought to person place or thing this stops the flow of energy to the thought, which voids the cycle of thought, at the same time letting the belief go. This enables me to stay living in the moment where everything is happening and un-happening at once.

Have no thought of the future, there is only now.

The teaching of Jesus keeps coming into my life. To me it seems sad that we, as a consciousness, took the message, crucified the messenger and called ourselves piously Christians. Having slain the messenger we have now glorified him and started the greatest personality cult in history of mankind, calling it Christianity. We filed the message away and now worship the messenger instead, even send 'missionaries' out into the four corners of the cellar and continue playing hard done by, remaining in the cellar. Who is really 'crackers'?

In applying these principles to my life, I overcame the need to wear glasses, just by being aware of what I was telling myself. What would happen, I would go to read something then start looking for my glasses, telling myself how much I needed them to read, putting them on and saying to myself, that's better I can see now. So I stopped saying anything, just finding the glasses and putting them on, having no thought to what I was doing. I stopped verbalizing, just putting the glasses on.

The result of this is that I have not worn glasses now for over two years. I can read the smallest print with ease, even threading a needle easily.

I gave up smoking the same way. I found smoking was not my problem, it was what I was telling myself. If I felt like a smoke, giving no thought or verbalizing the need to smoke, but continuing to smoke regardless, in a short time I found I never felt like a smoke. So I stopped smoking altogether within one week, knowing I would never smoke again. I choose never to wear sun glasses, allowing my eyes to adjust to any glare out there of their own accord, which they are quite capable of.

Have no thought of catching an illness - it is impossible.

The same with sun cancer - it's not the sun that causes the cancer, it's the belief that the sun creates it. A belief in two powers. My thoughts interfere with the flow of life. Giving no thought to anything allows my true self to shine through and allows my life to flow freely.

Thoughts held in mind produce of their kind.

When I was seventy years old I was working at a spiritual retreat with a man called Bill who was ninety years old. We were cleaning out the gutters on a high roof house on the side of a hill. We were both climbing up and down the ladders all day, and come three o'clock and Bill said, 'By jove, I think we will knock off. I tell you what Richard, I will sleep well tonight'. He told me that he never ever tells himself that he is tired. I practice this now, and it is an amazing example of how a simple 'no thought' or not verbalizing the thought enables the body to perform much better.

Have no thought of making a mistake - there is no such thing.

I now know that thoughts set up belief systems, which will always have a fear base. What causes this fear at a deep level is that

I separate myself from the Oneness - I go into duality. My thoughts at this level use up a lot of energy, my vibrations change and I operate at a lower frequency level, which results in me living in duality. I then self destruct, which in turn makes me receptive to catching illness coming from the mass thought , which believes sun causes skin cancer, heavy lifting causes back problems, mosquitoes sting. It's the fear of starving to death that kills, not the lack of food. I now know there is not one single disease that can affect me when I rise beyond the extremely low frequency of fear. The basic issues I need to deal with are thoughts based on beliefs and fear.

There is no such thing as person, place or thing, we are pure consciousness. What I see out there is an expression of my imagination.

Knowing all this, it is easy to see how all the symptoms in the body are manifested, by knowing what caused them in the first place, for man may know cause but never understand effect. So it's important to deal with them at the conscious level where they will not occur again.

It seems to me now that what thoughts actually do, besides using a lot of energy, is to change my vibrations to a lower frequency, this in turn destroys my immune system allowing toxins to build up in my body, which in turn blocks the flow of life. So it is futile to try and fix the symptoms.

'Little Tommy came and put an egg on the table. 'Look what I found mummy', he said, and as he spoke the egg rolled off the table and broke, 'Oh Tommy how can I fix that broken egg now?'

'I know how to fix it mum', he replied.

'Tommy please go outside and play while I fix the egg.'

A little while later Tommy came and put another egg on the table, which then rolled off and broke on the floor,

'Oh Tommy, now you have broken another egg.'

'I know how to fix them mum'.

'How could a little boy like you know how to do that?

'Easy mum. We will make the table level so they don't roll off.'

'Oh Tommy you are so clever.'

The most important and direct reason why mankind should comprehend the way the creator works in this respect, is because this book is written to demonstrate that man cannot violate God's orderly, rhythmic process of Nature without paying a price which is equal in measure to the violation.

I visited my friend Evelyn who had moved to a new area to live. She was telling me one of the main attractions of the area was the abundant supply of fresh food markets held every weekend. I pondered why she could not see that her need for fresh vegies was still a part of her life, I thought she had woken up to the fact that the *need* for a good diet of fresh food created a lack within. But no, it was *me* who hadn't woken up - another example of the 'mirror, mirror on the wall' reflecting all.

I have realized that, not only must I clean my body as part of my daily routine, but even more so I should 'hose out' my mind on a daily basis and replenish it with the highest and purist thoughts of inner thinking. It's not important what goes into the mouth but more important what comes out of the mouth. My father who had wonderful wisdom, said to us nine children one day, 'Gather around you blokes and let me tell you how simple life is. If we think good or God thoughts, that is all there is to life. If you want to exercise, deep breathing will suffice.' It has taken me fifty years to realize the truth in what he said.

Have no thought for suffering, for this causes separation.

This is the beauty of recognizing oneself in the reflection, for it's a wonderful means of letting go and voiding the cycle.

And so live in the now.

The most potent toxins I can ingest into my body, are fear, anger, frustration and the like. If I put a lot of emotion and thought with these I create a strong force that creates blockages and restrict the flow of life and so destroy the body.

Everything in life is made up of cycles, and each cycle is a complete lifetime in itself. From the microscopic to the macroscopic the same principle applies. My body vibrates at about fifty cycles a minute and electricity vibrates at fifty cycles a second. In breath compresses and is alkaline in content: out breath radiates and is acidic in content. If I hold onto thoughts, acid builds up in the body causing blockages and allowing illnesses to flourish. It is important that the alkaline and the acids always balance each other.

To give thought to a good diet is to give it power, which has a balancing effect of creating a fear within of being unwell. This in turn drains my energy which in turn alters my vibrations. To express who I truly am I now know the food I must partake of comes from within my beingness. This is good thinking and good living. As Jesus said, *I have food you know not of* .

This principle applies to any person place or thing. The result of doing this is a reversal of the flow of energy through my body, allowing it to express more fully who I am. There is much more to be got from within oneself than from without. As I create with the power of my imagination I have more to give, and re-give.

Have no thought of a thief, there is no such person.

My body of itself has no needs or wants, so if I let it express what I have already created within, without thought, reason, or purpose, life seems to flow more freely. I have a clarity of mind and a minimum of mind chatter.

I suffered from constipation all my life, having to continually take laxatives. A few years ago I decided to let go and let God, so with no further thoughts about how my bowels worked, I now experience regular bowel movements twice a day.

Have no thought of medication, they are all placebos.

I feel I am here this lifetime not so much to enjoy the abundance, but to give and re-give of that abundance coming from within. To me this is Love.

It is amazing how things *don't* happen in my life when I give them no attention (no thought). When I give no thought to the reflection, I realize what I am seeing is an aspect of my own self which has got nothing to do with the person out there but is an issue that I need to deal with at an inner level where the cause is. At this level I can deal with it so that it doesn't occur again.

Have no thought of love. I AM LOVE.

My body is inanimate. All the organs in my body are vibrations reflecting my consciousness this includes the heart – chakras – DNA etc, they have no substance of themselves. This body has never lived, therefore it can never die, the spirit lives on. Therefore this means the body of itself can have no feelings or discomfort. It is animated by my consciousness and is a reflection of my state of mind. Whatever state my consciousness is experiencing will be reflected in the physicality of my body. This also applies to everything else I see 'out there'. If the light is shining brightly from within me it lights up everything out there. The same thing applies when I am feeling down - the world out there is down. I take full responsibility for everything that is happening in the universe which is inanimate, having no life at all – no energy, it is only a reflection of mind, God in motion, pure consciousness. It is un-happening as fast as it happens in the Oneness of all. There is only one energy force in creation and that is mind, pure consciousness. There is no past or future, only the here and now. Eternity is now.

Have no thought for God. I AM God.

As I chop wood and carry water (which I call my daily chores)without rhythm or reason, giving it no thought or purpose but expressing my action with joy and ecstasy, I seem to have an unlimited amount of energy and a clear mind. To me this is the giving and re-giving of love, where I seem to have an unlimited amount to give without attachment. To me this is a true state of Being, which is to Be and not to have. I call it living in Love. The concept of *have* was established by survival thinking in opposition to the natural state of Being. To *have* means to be incomplete. Only a state of incompleteness can feel want. To live a life where fear and lack are experienced in any way is but death by degree. To need anything is false.

Have no thought of possessions. I have an abundance.

When I feed my body on the desires outside myself such as love of another, or the joy of a new car, I may think that the joy comes from these and so I create a big hole of lack within myself. The degree that I love another is the degree that I don't love myself. This breeds fear and frustration, which is far worse than any food that I might ingest, particularly when I add emotion (energy in motion) to it. The beauty I see in the rose is not in the rose but is a reflection of the beauty within me. All good things in life come from within me in the Oneness of it all. I must live inside out and see with inner eyes. The universe is within me. I may experience pleasure from the material world, but I can only experience happiness from within.

Have no thought of money. My supply comes from within.

For a long time I have been blind and could not see, now that I have awakened to the dream, I can see where the truth is setting me free. So much of what Jesus spoke about in The Sermon On The Mount, referring to the surrender of possessions as a prerogative to enter the Kingdom of Heaven, I sadly misunderstood: I thought they were material possessions, and money. The possessions in question are my fears and belief systems which oppose the Truth. Fear is the major 'possession' I am reluctant to give up.

Have no thought of helping another person,
for they are an expression of myself.

It is these fears and beliefs that are the cause that create material possessions. Living in the here and now I must always look for the cause of what is happening, never at the effect. To have no attachment to what I have created allows my life to flow freely. The need to *have* anything in this life is to do with holding on, which has a fear base. Thoughts that are fear based have a greater potential to manifest than otherwise. The less thought I give those fears the less power they have, so, 'give it no thought' for nothing matters.

Have no thought to what you put in your mouth,
only what comes out of it.

I have learnt that it is impossible for any man to know or understand any person place or thing, or the effect world out there (the material world). Therefore it is impossible to fix problems out there. First I must know myself, to look to the cause from within and change it from there. If I see something different 'out there' and I don't like it, or would like to change it, I know how to do this. First, knowing that I created it, then giving the something out there no thought or attention. By coming back to the Oneness, knowing what I am seeing is a expression of my imagination. The only way to change the reflection is to change the cause of the reflection, which is in my consciousness.

We live in a mirror imaged thought wave universe where we make believe that which we choose to experience, we then believe what we have created is real.

To think I can help another person place or thing, is my choice to separate myself by judging another.

You may ask what is a mosquito, when I release all judgement nothing will have a name, such as person place or thing – so how can I describe what my eyes see out there, the answer will always be I can only see a expression of my own imagination.

CHAPTER 6
WHO AM I

Soul – mind are One. mind is electric, the Soul is the expression of mind, my soul is me. I (Richard) live in a mirror-imaged thought wave universe where I and the Father are One. I AM a divine immortal invisible soul centered in a physical body made up of thought waves of motion. This body I call Richard is never created, only the 'idea' of Richard is. He (Richard) is within, and is the ONENESS of all there is.

Have no thought of death the body continually renews itself, moment by moment.

This is not a created universe; it is a creating universe, and that which is being destroyed exactly balances that which is being created. There are not two minds, two forces, two substances nor two things in the universe. Separateness and separability are impossible in this universe of the One Supreme Being. The appearance of separability belongs to apparent motion (dream world) and not to substance. All apparently separate things are functioning mechanically as the body of the One Supreme Being, and all apparently separate minds are thinking His thinking. They cannot do otherwise. The time has come where I must know where God is at every moment in respect to myself. I must completely understand how God controls every action and desire of all living things, from man to fungus cell, or from galaxy to electron. I must realize that where motion is it is centered by stillness and that stillness is its cause, which will be at ninety degrees to that motion. This is where God is, at the center of the fulcrum, as being at the center of the cyclone.

Have no thought of old age. There is no such thing.
I am living and dying simultaneously.

The only way that I can find peace and happiness is to discover my unity with my Creator. My greatest awakening will come with the realization that I AM all men (this includes women too). I have been given my ability to give and re-give all that back to the Oneness from whence it came. This allows the cycle to be voided so that I have more to give.

I liken this to milking a cow. I was brought up on a farm where we had four to five milking cows. There were nine children plus mum and dad, and at odd times we had to rely on one cow only for milk. So, in order to get enough milk we would milk the cow three times a day. The more often a cow is milked the more milk it gives. This law applies to myself also - the more I give the more I have to re-give.

On a recent trip to Ohio in America I experience a major triggering effect for me to awaken when I perceived the difference that exists between the black man and the white man. I saw the differences in living standards and values of white and black and the separation that is brought about by man seeing the differences in his fellow man. I have been experiencing an enormous amount of sobbing within the pit of my stomach, a feeling of shame that needs to be released as I let go within. My eyes are being opened and I can now see where I could not see before. I was blinded by the dream.

The universe is within man himself.
So to heal the universe, man must first heal himself.

What this is opening me up to is the ability to see myself in all creation as a reflection of GOD. WHO I AM.

For me to come to grips with that, what I am honestly seeing is *myself* in every created thing, and I know that I am that person, place or thing. All I have created is perfect, whether it is the ocean, violent storm, forest, black man or white man, or the flower in the garden. I can know the divine balance and abundance in all creation. I now see with inner eyes that everything is an expression of itself, the Oneness of it all. With this awakening to the dream, I have chosen to be honest with myself and to see with inner eyes only. I now know that I have never experienced love.

Looking back in hindsight to a trip to India to see Sai Baba, I remember an incident that occurred to me that pushed my buttons.

On my first day in India I boarded a train for Bangalore and had the compartment to myself for the first part of the journey. We had begun to move when I heard a noise under the seat, and looking down I saw a young man slide out. He had no legs and only one arm, which he extended to me palm up, begging. He had swept the carriage floor clean with a bit of bush. The beggar had the most radiant smile on his face that I have ever seen on any man, but I turned my back on him, refusing to give him anything, as I had been warned by many people not to give to beggars as they make a living from it.

I have realized since that what I saw on his face was a reflection of a childlike beingness of pure love shining from my own self. I now know I was the beggar controlled by my own stupid ego self. Every creating thing in this universe is self – created – and that SELF within each creating thing is GOD.

The greatest miracle that can happen to me is the discovery of my own Self, and my oneness with all other men. To find who I Am is for me to be able to identify myself in everything that is reflected out there - a mirror image of my own imagination, this is another example of like seeking like, which is the driving force, of creation.

I know that everybody out there knows all that I know. And I know everything every body knows I know.

When I am very honest with myself, I realize the universe is within me, and what I see out there in the material world is a clear expression of my imagination.

I now know all the conflict and suffering I see out there is caused by me, Richard, being separate from the creator within.

So knowing the cause of suffering enables me to be able to cure the issues I notice out there.

CHAPTER 7
INNER THINKING

Mind (consciousness) is the universe. It is all that is, ever was or ever will be. It is the seed of the universe. In the seed of the universe is the whole of the universe. The substance of universal mind has no beginning, no ending and no bounds. It is all intelligent, all powerful and all present. God and mind are One. The cause of all effects is dimensionless. Cause is existent, where effect is an illusion of existence. It but appears to exist. The force called 'thinking' which impels mind into concentration and decentralization in sequence is the only energy of the universe. There is no other energy. The universe is mind only. ...W Russell

Mind - soul are One. My soul is me. The soul is the desire quality of mind with which to create bodies to manifest idea. The mind expresses its creative desire through soul as pulsations, cycles, vibration, frequencies – as balanced opposites such as male, female, plus and minus and so on. The in breath, compression, half the cycle, is centripetal, masculine gender, and alkaline in content. The out breath is centrifugal, radiating, feminine gender, and acid in content.

To give thought to person, place or thing, is to see the reflection of motion which is seeing duality. This is the illusion.

The inner mind (consciousness) is divine mind. The inner mind of man is tuned to the higher speeds of ecstatic thinking, and is electric.

When I am creating with inner thinking and working with God, I have found that God will work with me but not for me. At this level I have at my disposal all the tools necessary - money, help, medicines, an unlimited supply of everything. But the powerful part of thinking with inner mind is my imagination. Inner thinking is subjective and dimensionless thinking. It is working with God, for the greater the imagination the greater the creation which is unlimited thinking, for God is at the center of my creations. It is at this level where I deal with all the issues that crop up in my daily activities. At this level my (Richard's) mind and God's mind are One; our vibrations are the same and actually 'hum'.

Know that that which you seek already stands before thee, you already have it.

I have noticed that when I am a bit run down, I can tense my foot and create an intense pain like gout, and if I tense my calf muscles a cramp results. But when I am feeling on top of the world, it is impossible create any pain.

Inner thinking is much more meaningful and powerful than outer expression that is dealing with thought - objective and illusionary. As I create within, all I desire to happen in my daily life appears. This is the creative half of the cycle. When I compress and fine tune my imagination with joy and ecstasy, this gives me an enormous amount of energy. The desire for like to seek like is the motivating force for creation to express. It is from this expression that I get all the energy for my physical body to chop wood and carry water.

There is no such thing as sickness, suffering or death. They are only beliefs, held in place by thoughts.

Through the day I express that which I have created within into the material world, not giving any thought, purpose or reason to what I am expressing - person, place or thing – and not even being concerned with the result of the creation. Doing it this way without thought, my vibrations remain at the higher frequency throughout the day. This seems to allow my life to flow freely. This is the voiding half of the cycle, where I re-give that which I have created so that there is no acid buildup in my system.

It is my consciousness (mind) that governs and controls the organs and health of my body.

All actions of all bodies are always under the control of mind which caused them. Bodies have no power to move through their own initiative, for they have no energy or initiative of their own. Initiative is extended to the bodies by the universal mind which controls them.

As I let all judgment go and shift my outer thinking with thought and a belief in two powers - to inner thinking with the creator within - there is a big shift in the level and speed of the vibrations takes place. This higher speed of vibration is much more powerful in creating, or in the healing of a symptom. This inner thinking encompasses the outer with the inner and thus there is no separation, which in turn allows the outer to function and life to flow freely with no blockages. As I work from this level of consciousness there can be no thief, murderer or sickness out there. These are just words I use to judge with. Taking this a step further there can be no evil, sin or sickness in all creation, for again these are just words of judgment, which become beliefs. When I see the beggar in the street I must not make the mistake as identifying as a beggar, and try to help him, but to see him as a soul experiencing this lifetime as being a beggar.

When I am balanced I cannot generate pain.

I feel I have reached the point where I can understand that all human conditions are make believe, and the human mind just *thinks* they are real. This belief resulted in my expulsion from the Garden of Eden. When I become convinced in my innermost heart that because God is infinite *there are no pairs of opposites*, I can say to the Master, 'I have overcome this world'. Then, I am back in the Kingdom of Heaven where nobody knows what health is because nobody knows what disease is. Nobody knows what painlessness is because nobody knows what pain is; nobody knows what wealth is because nobody knows what poverty is, and if one does not know what health and wealth are, how can one know what their opposites are? There is nothing to make comparisons; there is just God, just spiritual being; perfection.

When I keep thought in mind I keep fear alive.

When my commitment is to powerfully completing a goal created from within the Oneness with joy and ecstasy, this is where I get all my energy from - to express the idea imagined. When I express that which I imagine, it is important to completely let go of all attachments to the creation. This voids the cycle which allows room for a completely new cycle to begin. Creating this way allows no loss of energy being held in the created idea. I have found this to be the most powerful form of meditation I have ever experienced. To void the cycle allows the energy to stay within my own beingness.

When I judge and see the differences in creation,
my body will begin to self destruct.

The inner mind of man alone can think in light. Inner thinking is ecstatic thinking. Outer mind thinking is objective thinking, which I see as referring to person, place or thing and is controlled by my thoughts. It is the desire of mind to express that puts form to thought. The real driving force to express is for 'like to seek like', and this is what makes the world go around. This is the real purpose of life - for one to find oneself within oneself. This is why I have relationships with others, when like finds itself within itself the cycle is voided and this allows ones life to flow freely. When man and woman come together as balanced opposites, the feminine and the masculine become as One. What happens at this level is that the vibration of others becomes the same as my vibrations, and this in turn brings us into the Oneness of here and now where we 'hum'. When I can see myself in everybody else, and everybody else within myself, I would say I am living *in love*.

My senses remind me of stuff I need to let go of to stop myself from self destruction.

Universal mind thinks in light and registers thinking in light, which is integrated into the idea of the thinking and suspended for a time in the lower octaves of light in the appearance of form. This means that when I think, using my inner mind with God and the Oneness, I operate on a higher frequency where all is One. This is subjective and dimensionless thinking. This energy and idea is eternally existent as cause, and must not be confused with its effect in motion which are but dimensions, and are expressed as thought, therefore non existent - only reflections I must let go of. All thoughts deal with the outer illusionary world of effect. While ever I hold onto them I waste a lot of energy. My thoughts see the differences in people, places and things and make Richard believe they are real, for what I am seeing here and now is the dying half of the cycle that has already been created. This understanding makes sense to what Jesus said, 'Have no thought'.

Whoever shall drink of the waters of earth shall thirst again.

It has been a shock to me to discover that when I see an enlightened being out there I realize that I am looking at a clear reflection of my own self. Even when I see a wealthy person I now see a reflection of that wealth within my own self. There can be no enlightened being out there. They are actors in my play. It's my expression which will appear to change the world out there for they reflect my true beingness. For I Am All. For me to be enlightened I would have to see everybody as enlightened.

When I take judgment out of my life, I eliminate all blame, there can be no love, joy, happiness, trauma, suffering, war, murderers or thieves in the material world. Everything just IS - there are no differences. Without judgment I will be living 'In Love'. What I see out there is a reflection of the love and joy which are within my self. This attitude applies to trauma and suffering also. What I see out there are all a reflection of suffering within me caused by my separation.

To see somebody smoking and I don't like the smell of the smoke is a clear indication I myself have not given up smoking, it is still a part of my consciousness. So I now deal with this at an inner level of thinking where I can fully let go of what I see out there instead of removing myself from the scene where it will reoccur over and over again. It is quite remarkable when dealing with another person this way, for the fault we see in them is within my one self as I deal with it from within, and no longer see it in them, it appears they have changed, when in actual fact I am the one that has changed.

No one harvests but from the seeds they sow.

An incident occurred in America last year when I was with my friend Spirio, who was negotiating with a black man, Charlie, to do some work for him. Charlie was unable to look either Spirio or myself in my face. We both tried to get him to look us in the eye, but he refused, looking everywhere but at us. It appeared to us that he had been so downtrodden in his life he felt worthless. Again my eyes were blinded; I could not see because of my thought sensing ego. After six months of pondering this incident, and now seeing with inner eyes, I know that what I was seeing in that black man was a clear reflection of my own self not wanting to look at my own self. I was the one who was downtrodden and feeling worthless, driven by my thought driven ego.

As I have awakened to the dream where there is no ego, my inner eyes are now opening and allowing me to see and identify immediately what I am seeing reflected out there, so I am able to deal with my daily chores knowing I have created all there is. I am no longer blind, my inner eyes can see.

Having good health has nothing to do with the body.

A few years back I was at a dinner with a lot of spiritual minded people, there was a young chap there by the name of Jackson Wu, who seemed a evolved soul. He was sitting across the table from me when the lady sitting next to me said to Jackson, 'Oh Jackson I would love to be where you are'.

'If you can see where I am, you are also', He replied.

To me this was a profound answer that I have often pondered, to make me realize that we are all One.

As I spend more time living within, I become less concerned with the results of my life. Also having no *reason* for what I do helps me let go attachments. The results are replaced by a rich full abiding peace and an alert mind, a peace that makes the present complete. I am beginning to notice other aspects and benefits of living within, such as when I take medication for some symptom in the body I know the cause is in my consciousness. I become aware, as the body responds to the treatment much more readily if it is in a rested state of balance. The consciousness itself must also be relaxed and at peace with the world.

Good health is a state of consciousness. The awareness of this fact itself is a healing process. When I am wide awake, my body is like the rippled surface of a lake or turbulent ocean. It is vibrant with waves. Those vibrating waves of motion are my senses, controlled by my thoughts. They are also my body. My body is made up of waves of vibrant motion. Light is what appears when God vibrates.

The degree that I let separation go is the degree that the quality of my life improves.

For a long time I have been misleading myself believing I have been thinking with my mind when I have really only have been sensing with my body. My brain also does not *know* anything, for it is but motion. My intelligence sends messages to other senses through the brain. My senses cannot detect balance; I use them as gyroscopes to keep in the Oneness. I must be unbalanced or uncomfortable before the senses will vibrate to tell my other sensed nerves that my body is uncomfortable or cold. The senses can only sense one half the cycle, the seen half.

When I create at the inner level of thinking I am not deceived by my senses. Also at this level there is no duality and separation from the creator (God), for God is at the center of all my creations. My senses cannot operate at this inner level because they know only duality and separation. To apply the law of attraction, which is of the ego world, is to get something for self. This has a balancing effect which creates a lack within. I call this poverty consciousness.

To have a *need* for anything it would have to be false, or to seek to have anything is to deny the creator within. As I give less attention to the riches outside myself, I realize those riches are within my own self. My supply comes through many channels but the source is from the ONE within.

For so long I have been leading the life of a miserable beggar (prodigal son) living in the dream, not realizing life has prepared a banquet and has laid a table for its children overflowing with the best it can give, its Self. Instead of partaking of this wonderful abundance, sitting down at the table of life and accepting its gifts, I have been crawling beneath the table, contenting myself with the crumbs of life. I now know my being is my sustenance; there is no other source of supply. There is no such thing as giving and receiving where I will love you if you love me. The old ways do not work anymore. I cannot get anything in this life, I must now learn to give and re-give all that I have without attachment to what I give, for the more I give the more I have to re-give.

The word forgiving should be rephrased it should be re-giving. I now know that everything in this life is free. Even money is created out of thin air, it's written down on a bit of paper, and I call it money. We cannot give to anyone individually without giving to the whole human race, nor can we hurt one human without hurting the whole human race.

I can get no joy or love from my imaginings. This life is not about gratification

Love joy and happiness can only come from expressing who I AM. I am not my expression.

To live in heaven is to see no differences, where all is ONE, where there is no suffering or sickness.

To live in hell is to see the differences, and suffer the consequences.

CHAPTER 8
GIVE IT NO THOUGHT

In the Sermon On The Mount, Jesus made several profound statements that have had a dynamic effect on my life. He said 'Give no thought to what you eat or drink', and 'Resist not an evil person'. Each of these statements is interlocked. If I give something no thought I do not resist it, or if I don't resist anything I give it no thought. So it all boils down to no-thing matters. This is what I am waking up to as I let the dream go, true perception is to have no judgment. All is perfect.

As I awaken to the dream, it has helped me to understand the cause of creation, and to understand the cause of sickness and suffering, as separate from the effect world (dream world). The shift in my consciousness has been amazing. I didn't realize the effect, and further effect, of letting go of all judgment. As I write this book my insights are being superseded daily, whereby what I have written in the early stages is no longer relevant, but I choose to leave the book as it has unfolded to remind me of how I am waking up.

I thought that judgment was the main tool of the ego, but I

realize now he has many more tools up his sleeve. For me to transcend the ego is much more involved than I thought; the ego is a controlling force in opposition to God. I can get to the bottom of how he uses these tools I will be able to eliminate the cause of how ego tries to control my life.

All thoughts held in mind about person, place or thing are fear based; it is the ego's main tool to control. Thoughts create resistance and this uses up energy, which lowers the immune system. To have no thought is akin to giving in. Every problem that I have is self created through beliefs and thoughts. My ego uses my senses to convince me and to make believe that what they are sensing is real. A thought held in mind produces of its kind - we live in a make believe world.

Another profound statement in the bible, made by Jesus, that has had a strong influence on my life is:

'Therefore I tell you, do not worry about your life, what you will eat or drink, or about your body, what you will wear. Is not life more important than food, and the body more important than clothes? Look at the birds of the air; they do not sow or reap or store away in barns, and yet your heavenly Father feeds them. Are you not much more valuable than they? Who of you, by worrying, can add a single hour to his life?'
… Mathew 6:25

I practice this philosophy now of giving no thought to what I eat or drink, and the body lets me know quick and lively if I eat something it doesn't like.

As I awaken I am having a good look at my purpose here on earth this lifetime. To awaken means to see things another way. This is what Jesus meant when he said, 'turn the other cheek'. So now I am having a closer look at the tools the ego uses, and particularly how he uses my thoughts to control me. When Jesus also said, 'Do not worry', what this indicates to me is to give it no thought. For it's my thoughts that create words and beliefs, these in turn form judgments all leading to separation and suffering. My outer mind deals with thoughts, and it is impossible to see other than my own consciousness, which is objective thinking - thinking in dimensions. These vibrations are of a low frequency compared to inner mind thinking, creating with love which is subjective, and dimensionless and a high frequency.

All matter and masses of matter are the bodies of thought. All matter is pure thought.

The ego uses thought to create worry and fear - attitudes which originate from giving thought to person place or thing, and as such my creations are built on sand. So now when I see my fellow man as a beggar in the street suffering and I have the urge to help him, I must pause awhile and realize there can be no such thing as a beggar, for what I am really seeing is a soul experiencing the life of a beggar, a totally different set of circumstances. So no judgment.

Nothing real is ever created.

The major traumas I see in the world, be they war, tornadoes, tidal waves, sickness or such, I now see as my own Karma. To me this means experiences that I have not let go of, even though they may have occurred many lifetimes ago. If I am honest with myself, I would have experienced being a murderer, thief, pedophile, rapist and many other things. All these reflections I see out there are issues that I have not let go of. It is baggage that I am still hanging onto, they are all still part of my consciousness, issues that I have experienced at some time or another. Otherwise I would not have noticed them. All held in place by fear, this in turn limits my flow of energy and holds me in bondage of separation, creating at this level I can never know love.

So now I am slowly beginning to grasp that words set up beliefs, which in turn make judgments, which in turn create separation, which is the cause of all suffering. This indicates that I had better 'shut up', otherwise I will cause separation, Oh my!...

As I become aware of the full implication and further effects of this line of thinking, it opens up a Pandora's box of coming to understand vibrations and frequencies, which are the basics laws governing how creation works. I now choose to let the word belief go from my vocabulary. This is a stepping stone to no judgment that leads to not seeing the differences; all is One. At this level I will be living in Love.

To create with thought is to create with fear at a low frequency, where I create in duality, separate from the creator within. This is the level that the ego operates from; this is the ego's world. Whatever I Create here will always be the opposite of intent, which in turn separates myself from my true be-ingness. Operating at the lower frequencies of duality all my creation will be separate from God, therefore of poor quality and of little value.

> *I must have no thought or reason for any reactions to what I see out there.*
>
> *If I thought for one moment that I could teach this stuff I am awakening to, I would know I would be back in duality, plus it would indicate that I have not really got it yet myself.*

CHAPTER 9
ON SICKNESS

My whole life is now dedicated to living the philosophy that I have written about in this book. I live it daily, and the result is I enjoy excellent health. At 80 years of age I haven't been to a doctor for twenty years and do not have a doctor, or the need for a doctor or medicines. At the same time I have a large amount of energy to spare. I see every individual in the world as being a practitioner, a reflection of myself; he has the ability to heal the world from within his own self (my own self). For it is the state of consciousness of the practitioner which heals, that is where God is, God is that consciousness where there is no sin, disease, or death. If I (Richard) use the word sickness, and try and cure the sickness (word) whatever the outcome of the cure, one thing is certain - the sickness will reappear somewhere else in the body in another form or symptom. For there is no such thing as sickness.

It is the state of consciousness of the practitioner (myself) which heals; a physician who can divorce himself from the *word* sickness that refers to the patient's symptoms in the body. This practitioner, in the state of consciousness, deals with the healing at the higher level of vibration where his vibrations and his patient's vibrations are as in the One mind of the Creator where all is One. The power he taps into here is unlimited. At this level all vibrations are as One with the Universe. At this level he has tapped into the most powerful force in all creation where there is no sickness. The human mind plays no part in any healing.

In the same way I take the word *love* out of my vocabulary. My mistake is that I look for love in or from some person. There I shall never find it – never. The love I find in a person is a counterfeit of love. I shall find love only when I discover it as the reality of my being. What have I got left to experience? This gives me wonderful food for thinking at a deeper level and 'letting go' of all the old ways of trying to understand what it's all about. The truth of the matter is that the human mind plays no part in any healing. So I must go within where all the answers are. So give no thought to love or sickness. They both are an expression of separation, a belief in two powers.

Recently I have noticed myself in the way I walk sometimes on the farm when I have to walk a fair way to do a job. My steps feel heavy and my shoulders are bent. Then, when I go into town and am walking down the street, my steps are springy and I have my head up and shoulders square. Why?

Sometimes on the farm my old ways surface, and in this case it was the word '*work*' that came into my consciousness; it was the thought of having to *work* that lowered my vibrations, this is a clear example of how easy it is to slip back into the old ways of living in separation. So give 'work' no thought.

True perception sees any condition, any act or person as being in its rightful place for learning purposes. Although true perception is still a step away from Oneness, it still is only a stepping stone. It stands apart to the dream, it recognizes separation for what it is - only error, not sin. Not one single crime would occur if the world released judgment. To judge health as better than sickness will call forth sickness because judgment is born of fear and what I fear I empower, therefore I attract.

The instant I think of one aspect as being of greater value than the rest, I give birth to its opposite as a reality to be experienced. There are no pairs of opposites in the world. Good in the world of polarities is only the opposite of Bad. It is as much based on fear as Bad. So what good will good do? It will fight bad. Attack calls for defense, so it goes on never ending. When I judge I live in a self created prison cell where the force holding the bars in place is judgment. The instant I release judgment the bars collapse and I step into freedom. There can be no part of creation any different from another part. For me to experience the Whole, I, Spirit. That which is still wholly Spirit is that part of my Divine SELF, which is aware of both the seen and the unseen, for one is an expression of the other.

In the starving nations of the world it is not the shortage of food is the real issue, it is the fear of death; of not having enough food. The same with the thirsty man. If he does not get enough to drink it is the fear that kills, not the lack of water. Giving the man water may quench his thirst but will not quench his fear, for the next time around he will suffer again. True perception would now look at (fear of) death, and look at what death really is, another one of the ego's tools. So give death no thought.

To heal is to change the perception of a condition. It is not the condition. Better I get the beam out of my own eye before attempting to remove the splinter from my neighbor's eye. When I do that, my neighbor no longer has a beam in his eye. The first step to the Oneness is awakening to the dream. The second step is true perception, which has the exact same effect, although it is still a step away from Oneness. It would identify with separation but is no longer a part of it.

The final step is to realize that it is all an expression of my imagination. This brings me to the greatest contradiction in terms – the place where the cause of the symptoms really is.

If I am honest with myself, my reflection has been created from a fear deep within myself, because I believe what I see reflected out in the material world can only be cured from within myself. The consciousness that created the symptom is unable to cure the illness. This awareness becomes clear to me as I cease to judge the spiritual world by looking out upon the human world. Rather, I come into an awareness of what the spiritual world is, through looking out from God.

'My kingdom is not of this world.' There is no way to judge the spiritual kingdom by looking at the appearance: I must ask myself

what is the cause of what I am seeing out there. It must come back to a belief that there is something outside of self, a belief in two powers. Sickness must be a creation of my belief: to suffer must be caused by beliefs also. Therefore it would appear that the sickness and the suffering is caused by a belief in two powers. I then come into the state of consciousness which knows that the organs and the functions of the body have nothing to do with my life, for it's the consciousness that governs the organs of my body.

To give a treatment, I must be in the state of Oneness, for the treatment to work.

Our senses are vibrating waves of motion and they sense only vibrating waves of motion

CHAPTER 10
ENERGY

The source of all energy in the universe is the desire of the creator to balance His expression of Who I Am. This energy is what powers all motion, there is no other source of energy. For this universe is the sum total of electric actions and reactions expressed in thought waves of two way motion. Which is the I AM.

Energy exists in Cause and is expressed in Effect, every vibration (cycle) is an an alternating electric current. This an electric universe.

Cosmic Mind makes use of motion to manifest energy. Energy is uncreated. Energy is and it does not become. It can only be simulated through two-way motion in opposite directions. Energy is a fulcrum, which never moves but which manifests itself by motion extended from its stillness through the two-way levers of gravitation which compresses, and radiation which expands that which has been compressed. Gravitation and radiation are not energy; they simulate energy by expressing it in motion. This is an electric universe and is expressed as motion, the faster the motion the greater the expression of energy.

The dead center of the cyclone is stationary, this is the fulcrum where energy is.

The dead center of the crankshaft of an engine is the fulcrum where energy is.

Energy will be found at the center and at 90 degrees to all motion. Motion itself is presumed to be energy. Motion expresses energy but the expression of energy is not energy.

Now, if the visible universe of motion is a universe of _seeming,_ the energy that generates motion and matter certainly cannot be sought or found in matter or motion. In other words energy cannot be found in the universe of effect, but only in the universe of cause, the Light of Cosmic Mind. Therefore energy is a quality of Cosmic Mind. Energy is in the Creativity of the Cosmos, not in the creation.

Electricity is the divider of all ideas into pairs of opposites expression of that idea which eternally appear and disappear and reappear in endless sequences to create a universe of seeming change in a universe in which there is no change

All energy is expressed as motion. The energy of thinking mind 'creates' a universe of apparent time and motion. All motion is expressed in waves or cycles

The force called 'thinking' which impels Mind into concentration and decent-ration in sequence is the only energy of the universe – there is no other energy, all motion is an expression of energy, but there is no energy in motion, only a potential energy. Energy itself is stationary and is at right angles to motion, which is the fulcrum for expression.

We live in a two way electric universe of cause and effect: cause is the unseen half the cycle, and the effect is the seen half. Because our senses can only perceive the effect half, we think it's all there is. It is impossible to create anything without creating its opposite, even though we cannot see the opposite.

Inner thinking divides the undivided Light (God) into two divided, unbalanced conditions, generating forms through motion in space and time. All vibrations (cycles) are mind-energy in motion, which the One Light of God centers at all times.

Every action – reaction in nature is voided as it occurs, is recorded as it is voided, and repeated as it is recorded

We appear to live in two totally different worlds at the same time; the material world, of apparent time and motion, and spiritual world, the unseen world, where all is one.

Everything is happening and un-happening at the same time. There is no time or motion. These two different worlds only appear to be separate. Each world is using a totally different type of fuel (energy) to function, yet each is in perfect balance with the other.

The spiritual world, the unseen world, is the real world where there is no separation. All energy comes from the still center where God IS, and has no movement. This energy will always be at right angles to motion, which is the fulcrum, where God centers motion.

For me to tap into this energy I must let the material world of reflection go, and become totally mind in motion. This means to give no thought or attention to anything outside of my true be-ingness, which is my Christ consciousness (the conscious mind of God within).

God is my individual consciousness, and therefore it is my individual consciousness that is creating, feeding, nourishing, supporting and maintaining my body in its health, harmony, and beauty unto all time. I am being fed, maintained, and sustained from within. My supply is unlimited.

It is time that man must realize that the key to natures secrets can never be found in the visible universe, it can only be found in the invisible universe.

Naught exist but God, man exists as one with God, but until he is aware of his Oneness, he is but a thought – recording image of God's imaginings

Life is a fast winding up of light -waves into bodies of visible matter, death is balanced unwinding of light – waves into invisible matter

To see any part of the material world is to see the illusionary

CHAPTER 11
NO THOUGHT

My purpose here this lifetime is to Find God, Know God, and Be God. Jesus gave some tools to help me do this. They are three statements that came from the Sermon on the Mount that have a profound effect on my life. They are, 'Resist not an evil person', 'Do not worry', and 'Give it no thought'. As I have fine tuned these sayings and go to the deeper meaning doors have opened rapidly

By not knowing where energy comes from, also not knowing what energy is, my eyes have been blinded by my thoughts. Giving thought that energy came from fossil fuels, food, motion, etc. is giving thought and verbalizing the thought that energy requires effort. It's the thought keeps matter in motion that drains the source of energy. It is where I create with fear and it shuts my eyes to the real unlimited supply of energy that is free to all of us from within. The whole world energy crisis can be related back to knowing what energy is and knowing how to tap into the source. For this to happen I must know what caused the world shortage of energy. I can bring it right back to one word, *separation*. Giving no thought to person, place or thing, allows the true source of who I am to flow through the ONE MIND of who I AM.

The discovery of truth is in the discernment of the false. You can know what is not. What is you can only be. The real will see the real in the unreal.

It even requires an effort to be ill, or try and stay healthy, when in actual fact there is no such thing as a sick body, a healthy or unhealthy body. For the body is only a vehicle to use to express who I am. It is inanimate. It will also tell me when my consciousness needs a treatment so that the Christ may flow more freely. 'Mirror, mirror on the wall.'

The best and most powerful way for me to do this is have no thought and thus tap into the unlimited supply coming from the stillness within, which is at ninety degrees from the motion.

I now know how to overcome all the problems in the world, and to solve every issue that comes into my life. All I have to do is change what I see reflected back to me from out there. This is my consciousness guiding me on my awakening, for I live in a mind and motion mirror imaged universe of make believe, where my senses deceive me one hundred percent, for I AM all mind which is God.

To have no thought has got nothing to do with person place or thing, it's letting all judgement go

All suffering is caused by the belief that there are two creators

God – Love – Balance – I AM, are all the same thing, just different words, these words define being and have no motion

CHAPTER 12
THOUGHT

Thought gives form to motion, which I call matter. Giving thought to what has happened gives it power to appear in the here and now, when in actual fact it has ceased to be; it is in the past. My thoughts hold in my consciousness what appears to be the material world, which I *think* is he real world. This I now call karma - all those issues that appear out there that I think are real such as wars, starvation, sickness and so on. These are all reflections of my past that I have not let go of.

So now I choose to give them no more thought. Giving karma no thought allows me to let go of duality and I come right back to living in the here and now where I am able tap into the unlimited source of the Christ energy. I am fed from within.

To give thought to matter which is apparent time and motion is to live in the past, for what I see out there has already happened. It's my thoughts that give it power to remain as part of my life.

Thoughts give power to beliefs, if I give thought to traffic noise, I will hear it. If I give thought to being overweight I will get fat, if I give thought to mosquito's stinging me I will get bitten. When I give thought to getting anything, I create a lack. And so it goes on. Thoughts are energy in motion, Thoughts create angry vibrations which resonate out into the universe. When I stop giving thought by giving no more energy or attention to the thought of anything on the outer, I stop creating on the outer. This is how I uncreate that which has been created. To understand the cause of creation allows me to know the purpose of life. This purpose is to experience separation and then to know that I am sinning, that I will miss the target. I will then know where God is in the Oneness. And like the prodigal son I will come home to the Father.

> *To try to heal a body is a waste of time, it's the consciousness that caused the symptom, so it's got to be healed at this level. The body can never suffer sickness, only the mind*

> *Have no thought for the welfare of the body, for it is inanimate*

CHAPTER 13
THE LAW OF ATTRACTION

The law of the creator's desire to express, gets it power from the driving force of, *'Like seeking like'*. This applies to all levels of creation, from the microscopic to the universe. It is important for me to fully understand the difference between how this law works on the outer material world and the inner spiritual world,.

Creating with the Law of Attraction on the outer will always create the opposite of intent. If I give thoughts and affirmations to my wants and needs, I will attain many possessions of the so-called good things in life, but a balancing must take place on the inner. Whatever I create on the outer I create a lack on the inner, which creates poverty consciousness within ones own self and in the material world. Working at this level, no amount of attracting will ever fill the lack created within. This law will always have a fear base of not having enough. It also requires energy, so the body must be kept in good condition by good food and exercise. This also takes time and energy. The result –I still end up lacking within. This has a domino effect in the material world as my consciousness is reflected from within me to out there, creating poverty consciousness in the masses, and creating wars, suffering, starvation and the like.

Creating on the inner requires a totally different approach. I call it inner thinking. Creating at this level, I work with the creator, knowing what I choose to manifest comes from within my own consciousness and not from 'out there', but it will appear out there as a reflection of my imagination. I have within me an abundant supply of all I will ever need in this lifetime. To manifest this abundance requires me to use my imagination with inner thinking, knowing the more I stay focused within and create at this level the more of my needs will be met. At this level my mind stays clear and my body is able to function more freely, thus using little energy.

As I overcome the poverty consciousness within my own self, this will have a further effect of overcoming poverty consciousness in the material world of my fellow man. The miracle of manifestation is not *what* is manifested, but *how* it is manifested by knowingly working with God. I feel this is what Jesus tried to convey to the masses when explaining the miracle of how he manifested the loaves and fishes.

I may have many channels of supply, but there can be only one source, that everything comes from within oneself.

I now know how to get rid of the beliefs that create the symptoms, by giving no thought to the symptoms

I must let go all concepts that knowledge can exist outside My consciousness, for the whole universe with all knowledge is within me

CHAPTER 14
GOD AND LOVE

My understanding of God is that energy force which is at the still center and at right angles to all motion. The center of the cyclone is where all the energy is, this is how God controls all motion by centering it. The center of the crankshaft of a motor in your car is where there is no motion, just pure energy, which is the same thing at the center of my being.

This is where all knowledge is, as in the hard drive of a computer, as I create from this level which is the fulcrum (pivot point) for all motion there being no energy in motion itself, only a potential energy. The expressions coming from this level are pure Love. As I express this love without attachments I will be living *In Love.*

The body of itself has no energy, all energy comes from the desire of mind to create with joy and ecstasy, the greater the imagination the greater the genius. There are no two things in the entire universe, all is consciousness, the One Mind. There is no beginning or ending in nature.

The balance in all creating things is perfect, God's love is perfect, for it is balanced. There can be no part of creation that is not perfectly balanced. The creator's one law is the 'Rhythmic Balanced Interchange' between sexed opposites. The material universe of seeming reality is motion controlled by intelligence and powered by desire. One may violate this one law to any extent they choose but to there own cost, or they may find the glory and ecstasy of working with the law and order that underlies their being when they at last see that Light which leads them out of the dark.

Each soul has to walk its own path. However, all roads lead to the same homeland. In truth there is no road to travel, for what we call a path is but the awakening of the soul from its deep sleep, we are homeward bound.

There is no beginning or ending in nature. There is only a continuity of life through cycles of action and rest. The senses do not inform a person of Nature's cycles, which continually flow two ways, through each other simultaneously, from zero to zero without ever exceeding zero.

I AM THAT I AM

INSIGHTS

Man has control over his actions.
But he has no control over the reactions to those actions.

The trinity is created by the creator dividing himself into two balanced opposite halves, each half being a reflection of itself.

The source of all energy in the universe is the desire of the creator to balance His expression of Who I Am. This energy is what powers all motion.

All matter does is express consciousness, matter of itself has no consciousness.

The universe runs on electricity, which is energy in motion.

All motion is caused by the desire to find balance in the Oneness. Balance can only be experienced when at home with God in the here and now.

Cause is stationary and unseen.

It's the consciousness that must be healed, not the symptom in the body, for it's impossible to heal a symptom.

There is one fundamental truth in all creation, and that is in the here and now in this moment.

There is one law governing all creation and that law is balance.

There is no joy, love or God at this level of consciousness, the material world – this is a world of make believe.

As our consciousness of ourself grows to encompass each other and all things, we will think, speak and otherwise act as the Universal One consciously.

I create everything in the image of my imagination.

To have a belief in anything will always cause separation from the creator within, or a belief in two powers, every belief creates an equal and opposite reaction.

Whenever I have a need or want in my life I will always create an equal and opposite reaction balancing effect of lack.

Whenever I give thought to person, place, thing or circumstance, I create cause which then creates a reaction, this separates me from the one creator to a belief in two powers where I lead the life of the prodigal son.

If I **do not** judge and stop seeing the differences, there is an enormous shift in my consciousness, and I stay at a higher level of vibration where God will work with me (not for me) on all that I wish to imagine.

It's not so much about seeing the reflection as letting the reflection go and to see with inner eyes only where there is no judgment.

Energy is in desire of mind and is expressed in motion, which creates the appearance of matter.

Matter is an illusion and is but a mirror that reflects qualities outside itself to simulate those qualities within itself.

All energy is expressed in motion, the energy of thinking mind 'creates' a universe of motion, all motion is expressed in waves.

What I identify with outside myself is ego, my lower consciousness.

Working from a higher vibration level I will see only the Oneness of it all, the I AM reflected. The vibrations at this level are of a high voltage and create a lot of energy to express.

A group of people working together will only speed up the destruction of man and the world we live in – because the group is a separate entity from the Oneness

Les my son was telling me how sad he is when he see his son Paul on the computer playing games all day.
So I say to him, 'Why don't you change the way he behaves.'
'How can I change the way he behaves?'
'Simple', I say to him, 'let all judgment go – see him with inner eyes only, see the divineness in him, and he will change his behavior'.

We cannot give to one individual without giving to the whole human race. Nor can one individual hurt another without hurting the whole human race.

Our senses are vibrating waves of motion and they can only sense vibrating waves of motion.

The material universe of seeming reality is motion powered by desire.

It is time that man must realize that the key to nature's secrets can never be found in the visible universe, it can only be found in the invisible universe.

Naught exists but God: man exists as One with God. But until he is aware of his Oneness he is but a thought–recording image of Gods imaginings.

Life is a fast winding up of light waves into bodies of visible matter. Death is a balanced unwinding of light waves into invisible matter. Compression – expression.

To see any part of the material world is to see the illusion.

When I know myself, I will know I am the other.

My negative thoughts are the most destructive force in the universe.

To have no thought has got nothing to do with a person, place or thing, it's letting all judgment go where there are no differences.

All suffering is caused by beliefs brought about that there are two creators.

I know the cause of cancer, and the cause of death, they are but beliefs.

I must let all my needs and wants go, that is the need to help another

– wanting to be more loving is self destructive.

The world is perfect, to see the perfection is to play the role of God, and be God. Where there is no judgment, everything begins with me and ends with Who I AM.

I live in a universe of absolute perfect equilibrium.

Have no attachment to motion – which is duality, with this attitude I am expressing pure divine Love.

The degree that I let separation go, is the degree that the quality of my life improves.

It is the thought that gives energy to the belief that gives it power to manifest.

To heal myself I must first heal the world – for the world is within me.

As I let go of judgment, I am beginning to get a feeling of inner peace, as my true beingness surfaces.

My body has no energy of itself - the degree that I believe and have faith is the degree that I restrict the flow of energy.

The I AM is not this body called Richard. The I AM is the conscious mind of all there is.

Every like and dislike that I have in my life will have an equal and opposite balancing effect.

It is my inability to see the perfection that creates the imperfection.

As I let go all judgment, all I will ever see that is different is a reflection of my imagination, this I know can have no reality.

The material world is a clear reflection of an image of my imagination, I keep these images in motion by giving them thought.

The degree that I believe is the degree I will experience it, this applies to sickness.

All creation is perfectly balanced, there is nothing to heal.

It is the thought that gives energy to the belief which gives power to manifest. So have no thought to sickness or death, they are beliefs only

As I let all judgment go I am beginning to get a feeling of inner peace, as my true beingness surfaces.

It is my inability to see the perfection that creates the imperfection.

If I accept the fact that I am the creator of all that is, all my creations must be perfect and in balance.

The degree that I believe is the degree I will experience it, this applies to sicknesses.

All beliefs pertain to duality.

My senses are vibrating waves of motion, and they can only sense vibrating waves of motion.

Action and reaction are equal opposites, they are simultaneously expressed and sequentially repeated in reverse.

Everything I need exists in this present moment.

I am not my body – I am not my thoughts and I am not what I feel.

Having a healthy body has got nothing to do with the body.

Any body anywhere is an extension of everybody everywhere.

Cycles are waves and waves do not begin or end - they repeat, but there repetitions have no end.

The key to maintaining balance is to stop seeing the differences.

I must stop *seeing* the differences instead of trying to *understand* them, for there are no differences.

There are no problems out there in the word; they are all within my own self: as I change the way I see the world the world will change automatically.

Resistance creates a reaction, which then creates what I resist – this takes energy.

To judge means to resist, which creates reaction, this blocks the flow of life, using up energy – what I judge cannot give a good performance.

The universe is not out there – it is within man himself – just pure consciousness. Expressing Who I AM.

My senses can only sense motion – it's my thoughts that supply my senses with energy to function: stopping the thought stops the motion.

Thought gives action apparent time and motion.

To get annoyed about anything is to set up waves of motion which then must be balanced.

If matter is in balance, it cannot move without losing its balance.

Its my thoughts that empower the differences – so give no thought to the differences.

Every action creates its equal and opposite re-action simultaneously.

When I stop seeing the differences, letting go all judgment, where living and dying are only an expression of each other, where there is no ending, I will be living in Love.

It takes energy to own or possess something.

Thoughts are what man uses to create the world of karma, cause and effect.

The body mirrors the condition of my consciousness.

I cannot help or teach somebody without a separation from God.

It is the re action that restores balance.

When one takes action one must suffer the re action – back to the world of karma.

Mind is matter in motion which is consciousness in motion, to try and balance that motion is impossible for it is only effect.

The source of all energy in the universe is the desire of the creator to balance his expression.

The reaction to love giving is love re - given.

All of our problems in life stem from our unawareness or forgetfulness of the fact that we always manifest cause by extending it into effect.

Electrically vibrating bodies cannot know anything, but can sense everything.

Conscious mind cannot sense anything, but can know everything.

That which you can sense you cannot know. That which you can know you cannot sense.

What God is, I Am. My Father – Mother and I are One. I am not alone, I am the universe.

Electricity is the divider of all ideas into pairs of opposite expressions of that idea, which eternally appear and disappear in endless sequences to create a universe of seeming change in a balanced universe in which there is no change.

If matter is in balance it cannot move without losing balance.

There is no knowledge, energy, life, truth, intelligence, substance or thought in the motion which matter is.

This universe is substance-less, it consists of motion only.

God is the Light of Mind. God's thinking is all there is. Mind is universal. Mind of God and Mind of man are ONE.

The unfortunate error of science lies in assuming that the power which belongs solely to the fulcrum of Light-at–rest is in the motion of the lever which simulates that power.

All motion is a continuous two way journey in opposite directions between two destinations.

Every solar body is forever, and constantly varying its speed around its primary. It varies it in each revolution by going faster for one half the cycle and slower for the other half.

Every action-reaction in nature is voided as it occurs is recorded as it is voided, and repeated as it is recorded.

Life is but are reversal of death – and death likewise is but a reversal of life.

This universe is the sum total of electric actions and reactions expressed in thought waves of two way motion.

I AM THAT I AM

www.ingramcontent.com/pod-product-compliance
Lightning Source LLC
Chambersburg PA
CBHW060356050426
42449CB00009B/1769